WITHDRAWN

KT-436-345

the art of breathing

The secret to living mindfully.
Just don't breathe a word of it ...

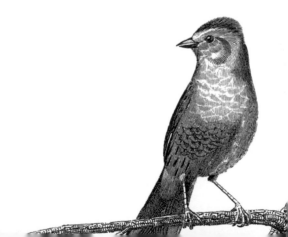

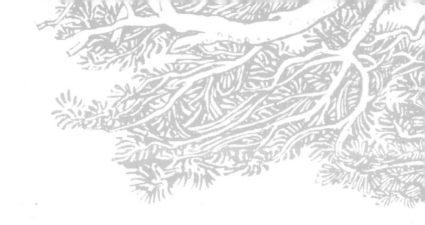

the art of breathing

Dr Danny Penman

Co-author of the international bestseller
Mindfulness: Finding Peace in a Frantic World.

Book design by Steve Wells

An imprint of HarperCollinsPublishers Ltd.

HQ

An imprint of HarperCollinsPublishers Ltd.

1 London Bridge Street

London SE1 9GF

This paperback edition 2016

3

First published in Great Britain by

HQ, an imprint of HarperCollinsPublishers Ltd. 2016

A catalogue record for this book is

available from the British Library

ISBN: 978-0-00-820661-1

Printed and bound in Italy

Dedicated to my wife Bella
and our two boisterous kids
Sasha and Luka.

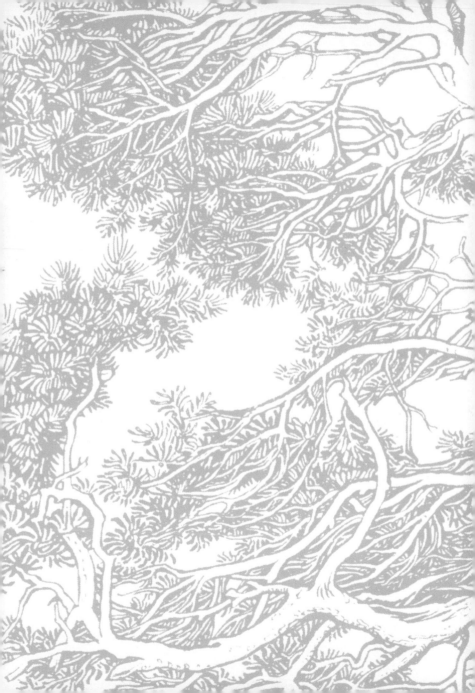

CONTENTS

Download meditations from
www.franticworld.com/breathing

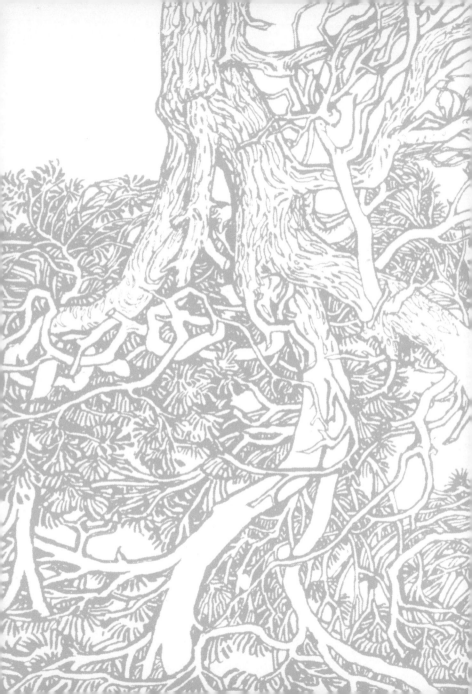

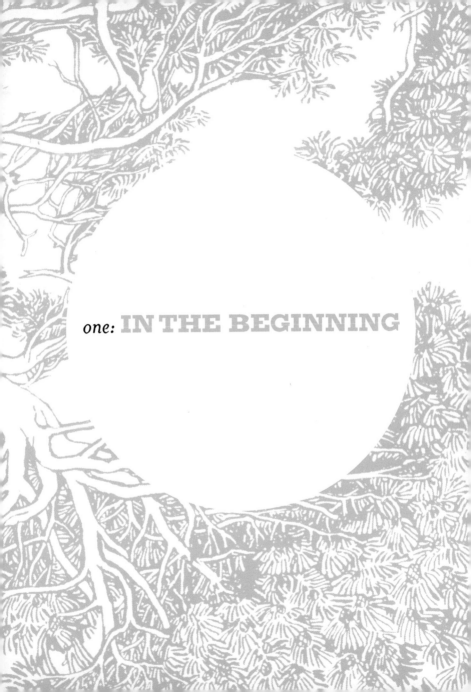

one: IN THE BEGINNING

Six paragliders are circling like eagles on powerful currents of rising air. Far below, a cluster of children gaze with open mouths as the giant parachutes dive and swoosh silently above their heads.

Then, suddenly,
something starts to go
wrong.

One of the paragliders is hit
by a powerful gust of wind,
turning the canopy inside
out. The pilot starts spinning,
spiralling like a sycamore seed
towards the earth.

After an eternity, the young
man smashes into the hillside.
He lies face down on the
ground. Broken.

But he is alive. After a moment
of stunned silence, he begins
screaming in agony. It will be at
least thirty minutes before the
paramedics arrive. And another
hour to reach hospital.

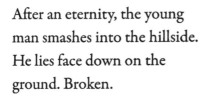

Alone, he knows that
he can't afford to lose
consciousness in case he
never again awakens. So
he begins forcing himself
to breathe.

Slowly. Deeply. With a
supreme effort of will,
he focuses his mind
away from his broken
body and onto his
breath. In. Out.

Inch by inch, the agony
recedes. Before, finally,
he reaches a state of calm
tranquillity.

Of pure mindfulness.

I was the young
man who crashed
his paraglider.

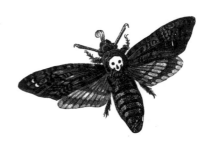

The art of breathing saved my life.

For thousands of years, people have used the art of breathing for equally profound effects on the mind and body.

Some have used it for relief from chronic pain. Many more to cope with anxiety, stress and depression. Some claim it led to spiritual enlightenment.

But I'm as spiritual as a housebrick ...

... so I use it to help me appreciate the bittersweet beauty of everyday life.

Your breath is the greatest asset you have. It's naturally meditative and always with you. It reflects your most powerful emotions and allows you to either soothe or harness them. It helps you to feel solid, whole, and in complete control of your life while grounding you in the present moment, clarifying the mind, and unshackling your instincts.

The art of breathing kindles a sense of wonder, awe, and curiosity – the very foundations of a happier and more meaningful life.

It grants you the courage to accept yourself with all of your faults and failings. To treat yourself with the kindness, empathy and compassion that you truly need, and helps you to look outwards and embrace the world.

When you've mastered the art of breathing, you will finally be at peace with yourself and the world.

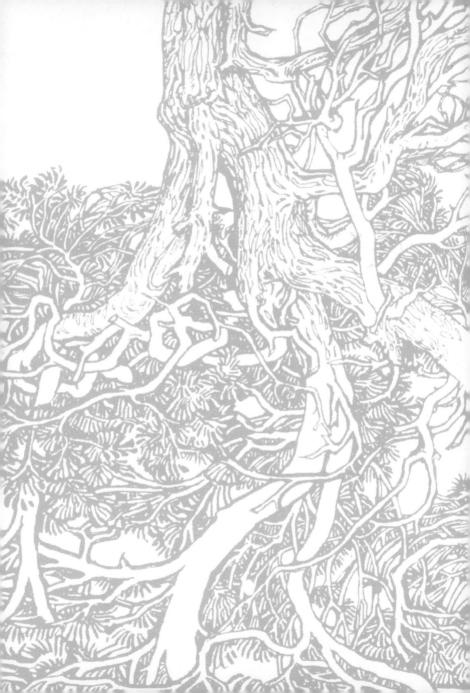

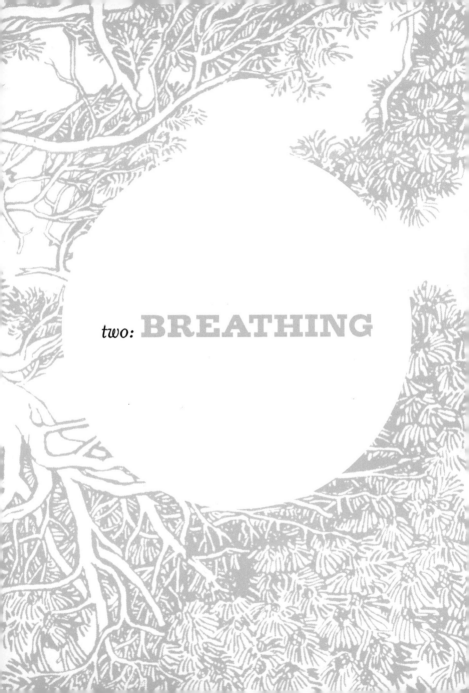

two: **BREATHING**

'As long as you are breathing, there is more right with you than wrong with you.' – Jon Kabat-Zinn

It all begins with your very first breath ...

Just after being born, imperceptibly at first, but with slowly building momentum, your tiny lungs began to inflate.

Nestling in your mother's arms, you began learning how to breathe. It wasn't easy.

A baby's breathing isn't naturally rhythmic. Babies breathe only when they need to, often with terrifyingly long gaps between breaths, not with a natural fluid motion.

As the weeks passed into months, your breathing developed its own natural rhythm. But, even now, you can soak up the rhythms of another's breath.

Lovers' breaths are entwined. Crowds breathe in harmony. Even the breaths of our pets can become entrained with ours.

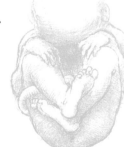

None of us are separate.

Although it feels stubbornly so.

You breathe 22,000 times a day. How many are you aware of?

Your breathing is so ordinary, so mundane, that its true significance can easily pass you by.

Lie flat on the ground with a cushion under your head. Place your hands on your stomach. Feel them rise and fall as you breathe in ... and out.

As the breath waxes and wanes, the abdominal organs rise and fall by 4 - 5 centimetres. This pumps oxygen and nutrient-rich fluids through the lymphatic system, flushing out toxins. The physical movement of the breath in the body also massages the liver, kidneys, intestines, joints of the spine, indeed everything, so they're kept healthy, supple, and well lubricated.

The breath is life ...

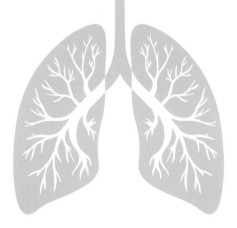

... on countless levels.

Your breathing both reflects and amplifies your emotions

Momentary stress causes the body to tense and you begin to breathe a little more shallowly. A shallow breath lowers oxygen levels in the blood, which the brain senses as stress.

Breathing becomes a little quicker and shallower. Oxygen levels fall a little more.

The heart begins to race. The brain feels a little more stressed.

IT'S A VICIOUS CYCLE

But there is an alternative ...

A gently rising and falling breath stimulates the parasympathetic nervous system.

You begin to relax.

Soothing hormones flow through the body.

These calm negative thoughts, feelings and emotions so you begin to breathe a little more slowly and deeply.

IT'S A VIRTUOUS CYCLE

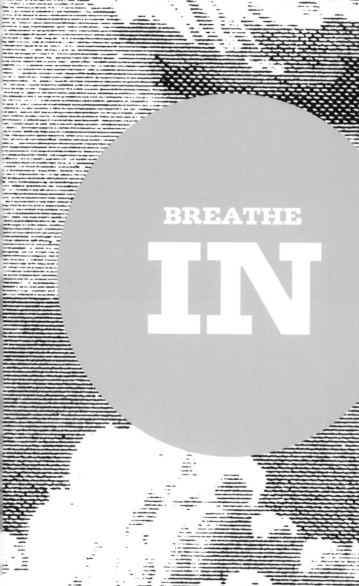

BREATHE
IN

BREATHE
OUT

When in doubt, breathe out.

Breathing relies on the big, powerful muscles of the diaphragm, the abdomen and the intercostal muscles that lie between the ribs. It is helped along by the smaller secondary muscles of the neck, shoulders and upper ribs.

When you are upset, anxious or stressed, the abdomen tenses and prevents the big primary muscles from working. Instead, they begin tugging against each other, leaving the secondary muscles to do all the work. But the secondary muscles are only designed to shoulder 20 per cent of the burden, so they become stressed.

If this continues, it can lead to chronic tension in the shoulders and neck, to headaches and fatigue, and to increasingly shallower breathing.

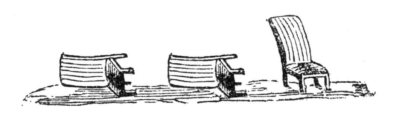

It really is as simple as breathing …

To breathe correctly, all you need to do is set your breath free. Mindfully submit to its natural rhythm. Feel the air as it flows in and out of your body. Allow yourself to relax into the breath's fluidity.

Feel your shoulders loosen and unfurl. Close your eyes (if you want to) and feel the ground beneath your feet.

If you feel anxious, distressed, unhappy or exhausted, then begin to consciously breathe in and out.

Take a long, deep breath while counting slowly to 5 in your mind. Pause for a moment. Then breathe out while counting to 7.

You can alter the speed of the counting to reflect the unique rhythm of your breath. Try not to rush things.

Repeat this 5/7 breathing until you feel more solid, whole and in control. You can come back to it as often as you like.

ONE

TWO

IN

FOUR — THREE

FIVE

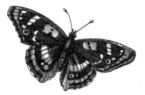

ONE — TWO

THREE — FOUR

OUT

FIVE — SIX

SEVEN

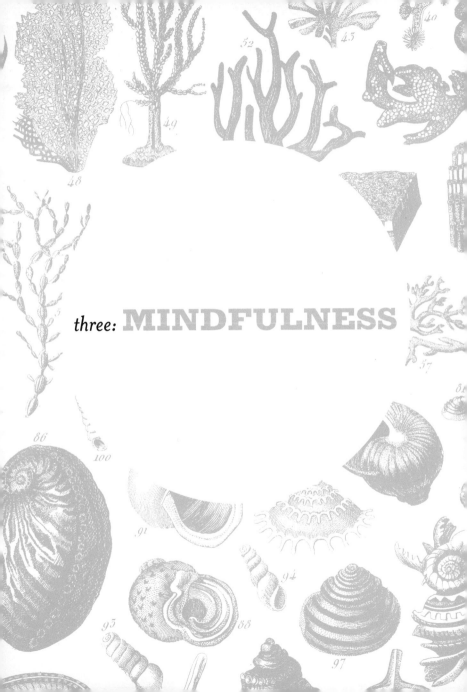

three: MINDFULNESS

The art of breathing lies in paying attention to your breath in a very special way. It's the heart of mindfulness and as old as meditation itself. You can learn the basics in just a few minutes …

… but mastering the art of breathing takes somewhat longer.

Breathing meditations are very simple but people often make them difficult and complicated.

Firstly, meditating in the lotus position is very uncomfortable. You can't meditate if you're not comfortable. Take a deep breath …

… and ask why the chair was invented.

Secondly, you don't need any equipment, mantras, incense, fancy bells, apps, or even a quiet room.

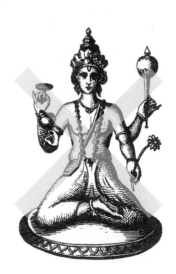

In fact, all you
need is:

a Chair
a Body
some Air
your Mind
that's It.

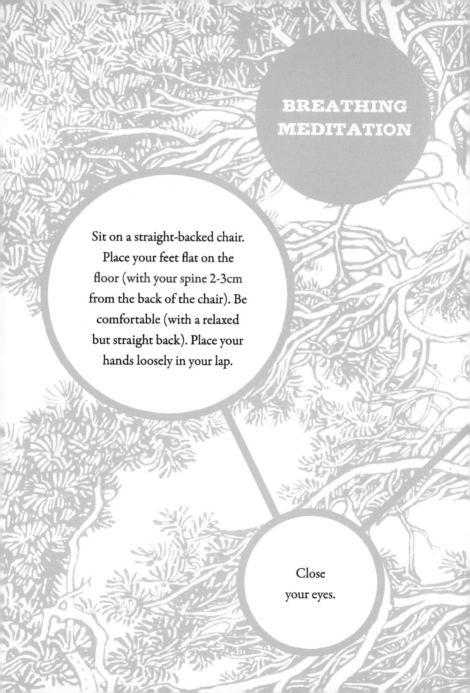

BREATHING MEDITATION

Sit on a straight-backed chair. Place your feet flat on the floor (with your spine 2-3cm from the back of the chair). Be comfortable (with a relaxed but straight back). Place your hands loosely in your lap.

Close your eyes.

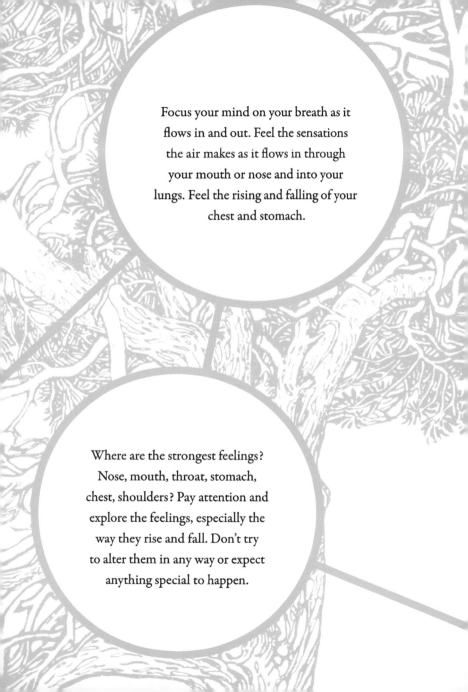

Focus your mind on your breath as it flows in and out. Feel the sensations the air makes as it flows in through your mouth or nose and into your lungs. Feel the rising and falling of your chest and stomach.

Where are the strongest feelings? Nose, mouth, throat, stomach, chest, shoulders? Pay attention and explore the feelings, especially the way they rise and fall. Don't try to alter them in any way or expect anything special to happen.

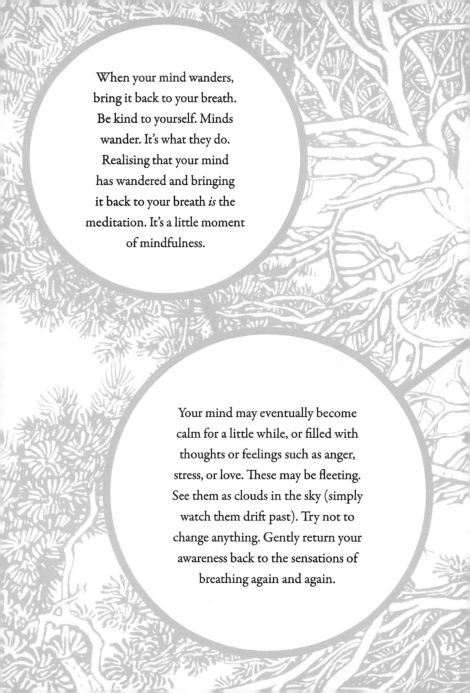

When your mind wanders,
bring it back to your breath.
Be kind to yourself. Minds
wander. It's what they do.
Realising that your mind
has wandered and bringing
it back to your breath *is* the
meditation. It's a little moment
of mindfulness.

Your mind may eventually become
calm for a little while, or filled with
thoughts or feelings such as anger,
stress, or love. These may be fleeting.
See them as clouds in the sky (simply
watch them drift past). Try not to
change anything. Gently return your
awareness back to the sensations of
breathing again and again.

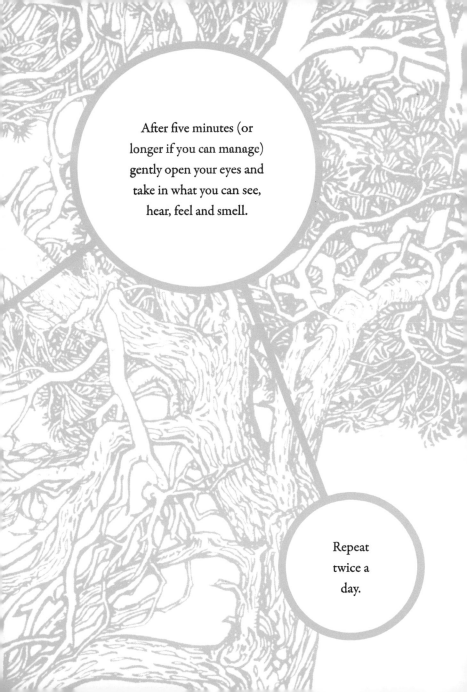

After five minutes (or longer if you can manage) gently open your eyes and take in what you can see, hear, feel and smell.

Repeat twice a day.

Did you feel restless and uncomfortable? Discover a few
aches and pains? Perhaps there was a long list of things
that needed doing RIGHT NOW, THIS MINUTE.

Maybe you had wild swings of energy. One moment
you were bubbling with enthusiasm, then suddenly ...
exhausted.

And the powerful emotions that swept you along –
the frustrations and disappointments, the feelings of
inadequacy followed by the bitter taste of defeat as yet
again you realised that your mind had wandered away
from your breath.

You probably felt that your mind was so chaotic you will
never be able to focus for more than a few seconds at a
time. What a mess ...

This is normal.

It's your first lesson.

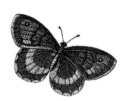

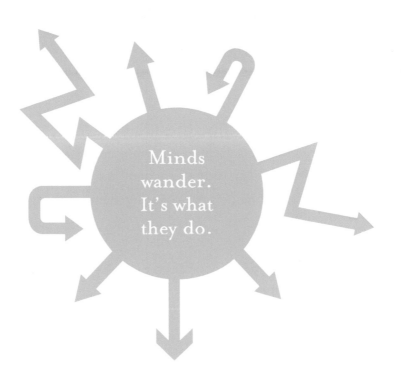

Minds
wander.
It's what
they do.

This leads to the central guiding
principle of mindfulness:
you cannot fail. Realising that your
mind has wandered away from the
breath *is* the meditation.

It is a moment of mindfulness.

MINDFULNESS IS
FULL CONSCIOUS AWARENESS

It is paying full conscious attention to
whatever thoughts, feelings and emotions
are flowing through your mind, body and
breath without judging or criticising them
in any way.

It is being fully aware of whatever is
happening in the present moment without
being trapped in the past or worrying about
the future.

It is living *in* the moment not *for*
the moment.

MINDFULNESS IS NOT
A RELIGION

Nor is it
'opting out'
or detaching
yourself from
the world.

It's about
connecting
and embracing
life in all of its
chaotic beauty,
with all of
your faults and
foibles.

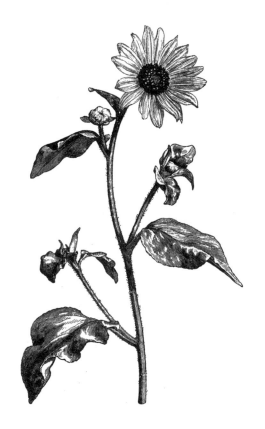

THE AIM OF MINDFULNESS IS NOT TO INTENTIONALLY CLEAR THE MIND OF THOUGHTS

It is to understand how the mind works. To see how it unwittingly ties itself in knots to create anxiety, stress, unhappiness and exhaustion.

It teaches you to observe how your thoughts, feelings and emotions rise and fall like waves on the sea.

And in the calm spaces in between lie moments of piercing insight.

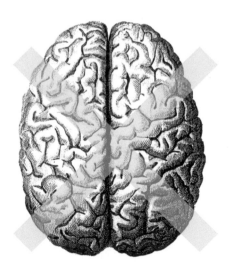

YOU ARE NOT YOUR THOUGHTS. YOU ARE THE OBSERVER OF YOUR THOUGHTS

It's a subtle distinction that's only perceived with practice.

Your thoughts are a running commentary on the world; a 'best guess' of what's truly happening. Often, your thoughts will reflect the powerful emotional currents swirling through your mind, body and breath.

Sometimes they are true, sometimes they are a frantic work in progress, sometimes they are wrong.

Mindfulness teaches you to take the long view, to put your thoughts, feelings and emotions into a broader context.

And when you do so, your most frantic and distressing thoughts simply melt away of their own accord, leaving behind a calm, clear, insightful mind.

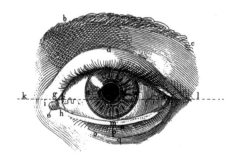

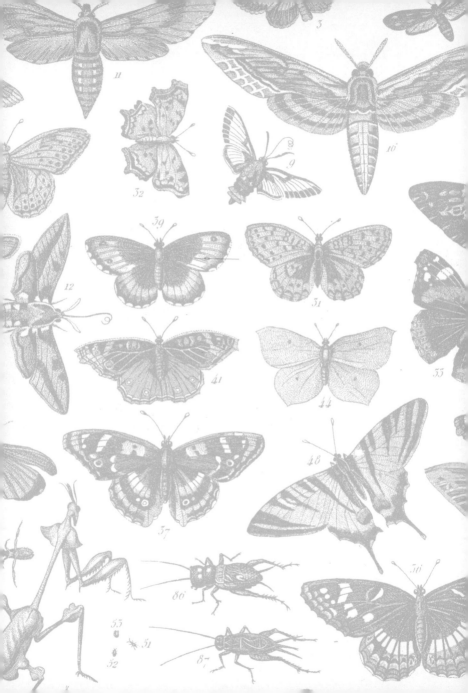

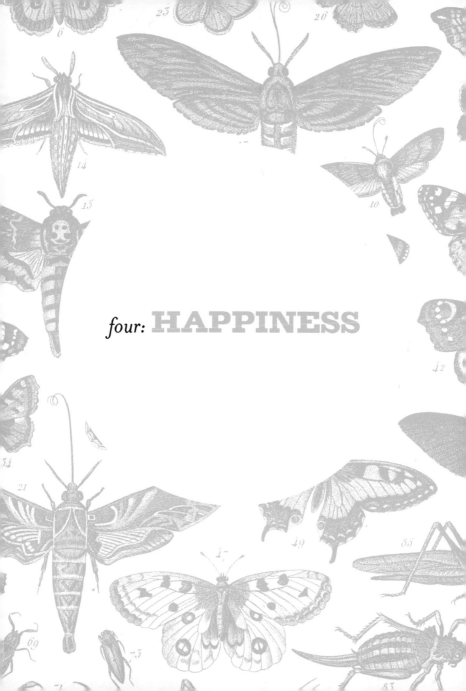

four: **HAPPINESS**

Happiness is fleeting whilst unhappiness
lingers.

It's called the 'Negativity Bias' and it's hardwired into
the very core of our being. It skews perception and
makes the world seem far harsher, bleaker and more
competitive than it actually is.

But life really is full of opportunities and pleasures.

It's just that the brain routinely tricks
us into thinking otherwise. Luckily, we
can redress the balance with the art of
breathing.

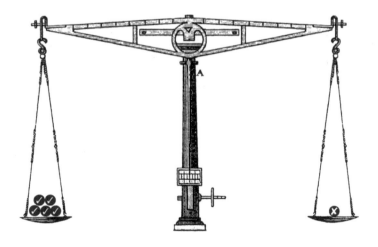

Nature compels us to avoid threats and seek out resources. It's one of the driving forces behind Natural Selection, but it comes with a powerful inbuilt bias. Far better to avoid threats, and survive, even if it means we fail to gain any number of rewards.

Instinct encourages us to assume the worst, to err on the side of caution, to live in fear and hide in the background.

The Negativity Bias ensures that it takes five positive experiences to balance a single negative one of equal magnitude.

This is a little dispiriting.

But then again, Nature doesn't care if we're happy but she does take a keen interest in our survival.

That's the point of Natural Selection, after all.

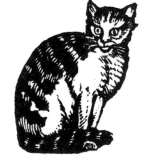

Thankfully, we are conscious creatures, so we can restore the balance and gain a happier and more accurate picture of the world.

It's no more difficult than periodically tuning into the breath while paying attention to the little pleasures of daily life. It means noticing the sights, sounds, smells and textures that surround you and soaking up the tastes and aromas of everything that you eat and drink.

It means giving your senses the attention they deserve while allowing them to intensify naturally.

And, while you do so, gently remind yourself that ...

... most of life's difficulties are only half as bad as they appear, while the good things are two or three times as intense.

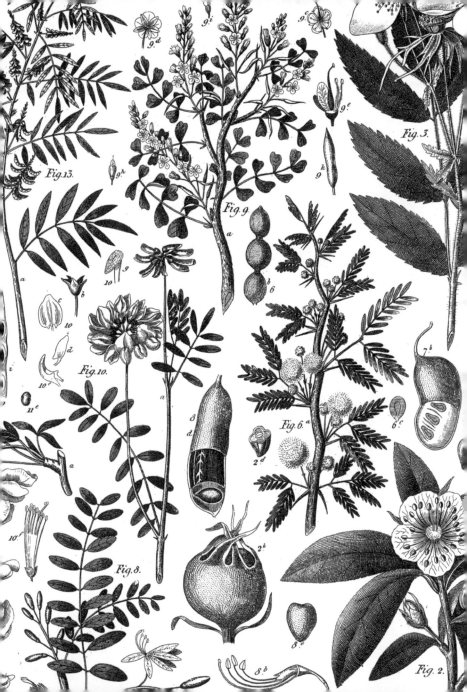

Fig.13.

Fig.3.

Fig.9.

Fig.10.

Fig.8.

Fig.6.

Fig.2.

Begin by
eating some
fruit

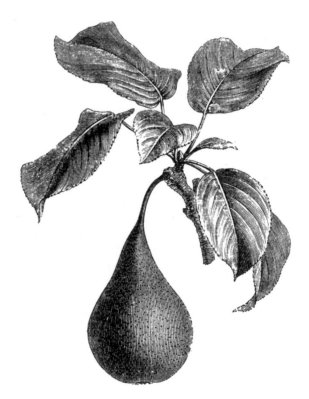

FRUIT MEDITATION

Choose a type of fruit that you haven't eaten recently (or even better, one that you've never eaten before).

Ground yourself by focusing on the rise and fall of your breath for 20-30 seconds.

Look at the fruit. Let your eyes soak up everything you can see. Is it smooth, furry, rough, jaggedy or shiny?

Inhale its smell.

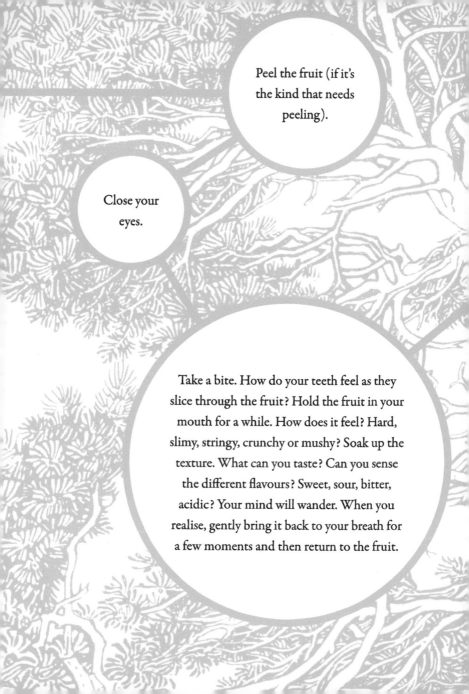

Peel the fruit (if it's the kind that needs peeling).

Close your eyes.

Take a bite. How do your teeth feel as they slice through the fruit? Hold the fruit in your mouth for a while. How does it feel? Hard, slimy, stringy, crunchy or mushy? Soak up the texture. What can you taste? Can you sense the different flavours? Sweet, sour, bitter, acidic? Your mind will wander. When you realise, gently bring it back to your breath for a few moments and then return to the fruit.

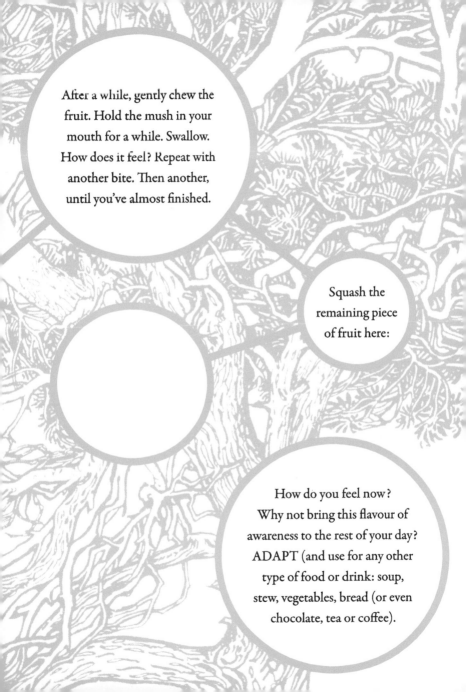

After a while, gently chew the fruit. Hold the mush in your mouth for a while. Swallow. How does it feel? Repeat with another bite. Then another, until you've almost finished.

Squash the remaining piece of fruit here:

How do you feel now? Why not bring this flavour of awareness to the rest of your day? ADAPT (and use for any other type of food or drink: soup, stew, vegetables, bread (or even chocolate, tea or coffee).

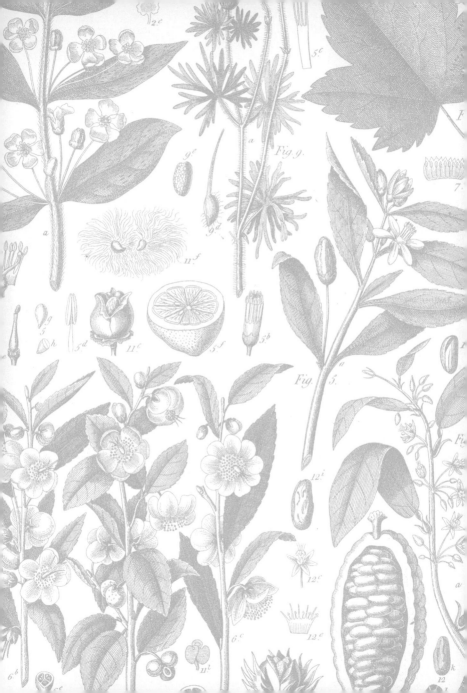

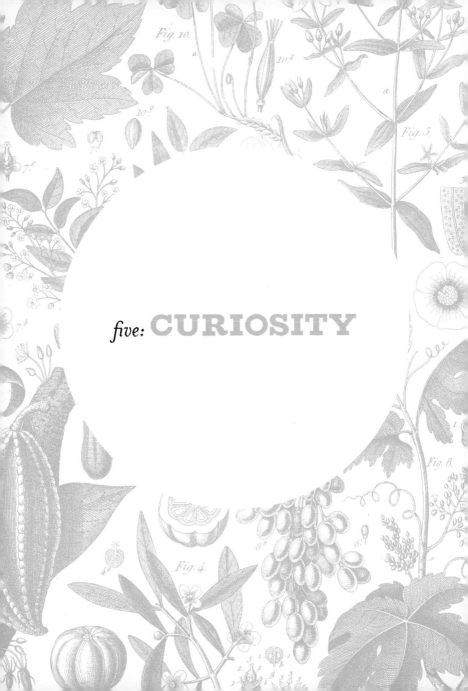

five: CURIOSITY

It's impossible to be unhappy and curious at the same time.

And around half of your life is ruled by habit.

They may streamline your life and free up time
and energy for you to do more useful and
interesting things.

But they can also become a trap ... quite a vicious one.
Habits begin wearing grooves in the mind and become
hardwired into your brain.

One habit triggers the next, and the next, so that whole
chunks of your life are run on autopilot.
Unless you're careful, they'll
control almost every aspect of
your life, including your taste in
food, clothes, music and even
your choice of partners.

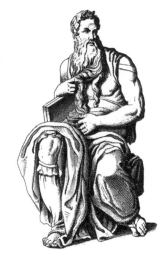

Habits govern how you interact with everyone around you, how you solve problems, conjure up 'new' ideas, and your entire approach to the world.

As Aristotle once said, 'We are what we repeatedly do.'

Habits can enhance limitations and trap you in negative states of mind. And the more often you criticise yourself, the easier it is to slip into the same habit the next time, and the next, and the next.

- What's up with me today?
- Why do I keep doing stupid things like this?
- Why can't I just do it?
- My life's a bit of a mess.
- I'm knackered.

One thought triggers the next, and the next, in an endless downward spiral.

It's the sound of your inner critic – and it's always with you.

Your inner critic is the voice of the Negativity Bias. And you're ushering it along by habit.

But habits aren't destiny, unless you allow them to be.

Habits arise when your mind is elsewhere.

They dissolve when you mindfully bring your focus back to the present moment. Observe your habits often enough and their underlying neural patterns will wither away to leave behind a calmer, clearer, more insightful mind.

So, when you realise you've been snared by an unwanted habit, or feel trapped by your inner critic, or suffer from anxious, stressful, bleak or otherwise negative thoughts ...

... do something they'll really hate.

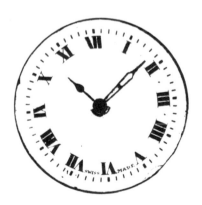

Take a few, gentle, deep breaths. Feel the ground beneath your feet ...

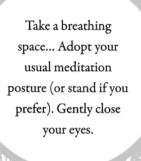

Take a breathing space... Adopt your usual meditation posture (or stand if you prefer). Gently close your eyes.

BREATHING SPACE MEDITATION

Step 1:
Arriving

Begin by noticing whatever is going on around you. Become aware of the space around you. Feel the ground beneath your feet.

What's going on in your mind and body right now? Briefly scan through your body and tune in to the most noticeable sensations. Don't try to change anything, simply feel the sensations.

Begin paying attention to the emotions flowing through your mind and body. Don't try to change anything, pay attention to their intensity and notice how they rise and fall.

What thoughts are around? Don't try to change anything. Simply observe them. Remember that thoughts are not facts.

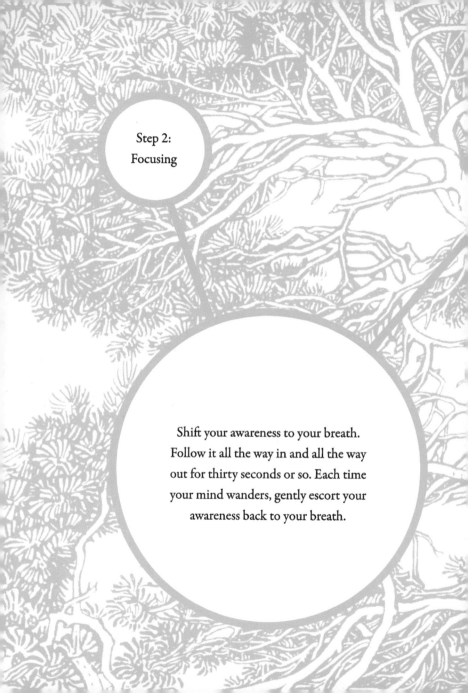

Step 2:
Focusing

Shift your awareness to your breath.
Follow it all the way in and all the way
out for thirty seconds or so. Each time
your mind wanders, gently escort your
awareness back to your breath.

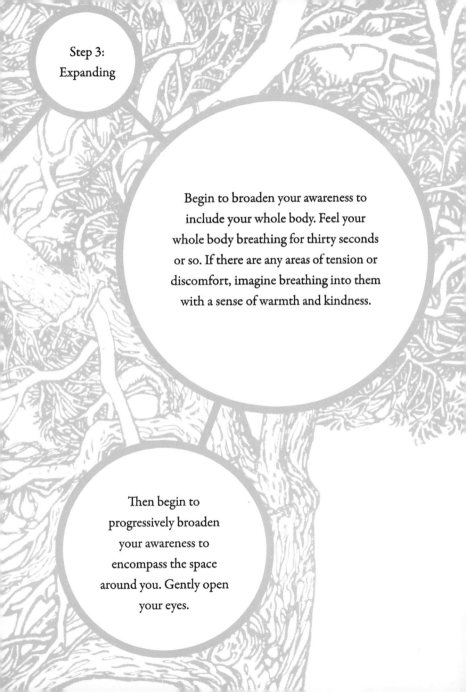

Step 3:
Expanding

Begin to broaden your awareness to include your whole body. Feel your whole body breathing for thirty seconds or so. If there are any areas of tension or discomfort, imagine breathing into them with a sense of warmth and kindness.

Then begin to progressively broaden your awareness to encompass the space around you. Gently open your eyes.

CURIOSITY KILLS HABITS

Things to break and do …

Habits are the mind's sheepdogs. Set yourself free by unleashing your curiosity. Do as many of the following as you wish.

Whatever you do, do it consciously, with full awareness.

Be Curious. Be Energetic. Be Alive.

Spend thirty minutes less at work.

Sit at a different table or chair.

Pick up a new book to get lost in.

Watch the sky for half an hour.

Take a different commute to work.

Stop every two hours and consciously breathe.

Go to the seaside, the countryside, the mountains or even the local park.

Switch supermarkets.

Eat something you've never eaten before.

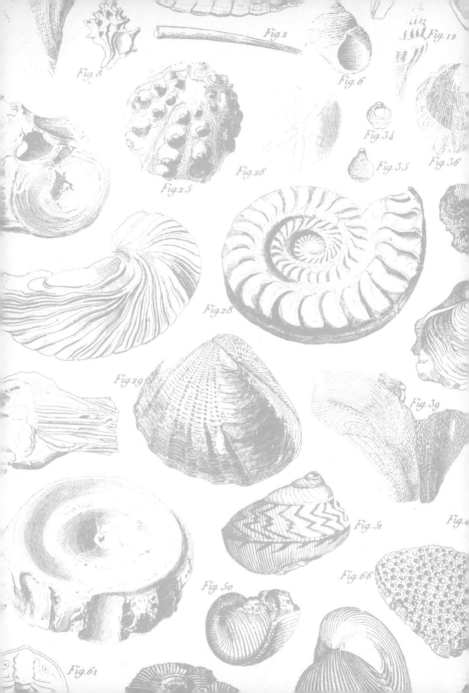

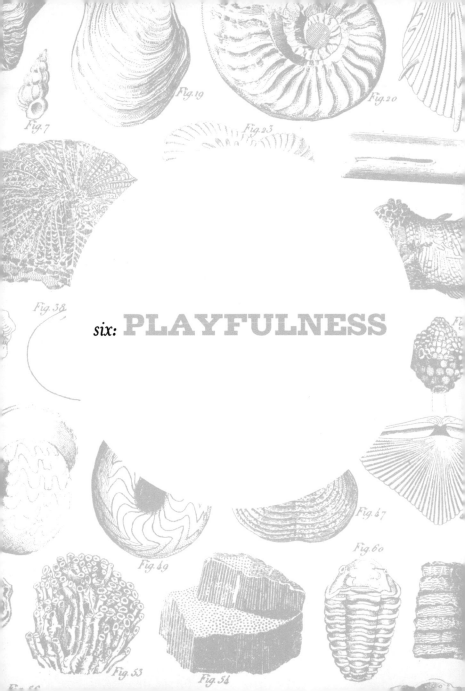

six: **PLAYFULNESS**

Fig. 7

Fig. 19

Fig. 20

Fig. 23

Fig. 38

Fig. 49

Fig. 47

Fig. 60

Fig. 53

Fig. 54

You'll probably spend thirty-six minutes worrying today (most people do). Why not go outside and breathe instead?

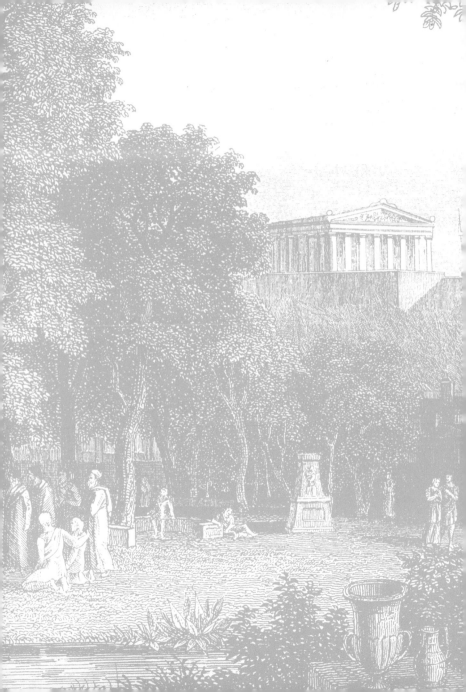

When you were a child, the world was a magical place.
You'd go to the park and collect pinecones and flowers.
Birds inspired awe and dogs were mythical beasts.

You could hardly make it home without your pockets
becoming stuffed with twigs, stones and other souvenirs.

Where did all that playful curiosity go?

nowhere

It's simply become paved over with expectations,
conditioning, and maybe a little shyness and cynicism.

It's time to breathe freely again.

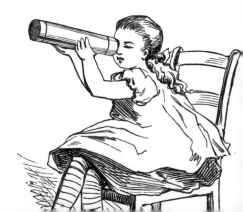

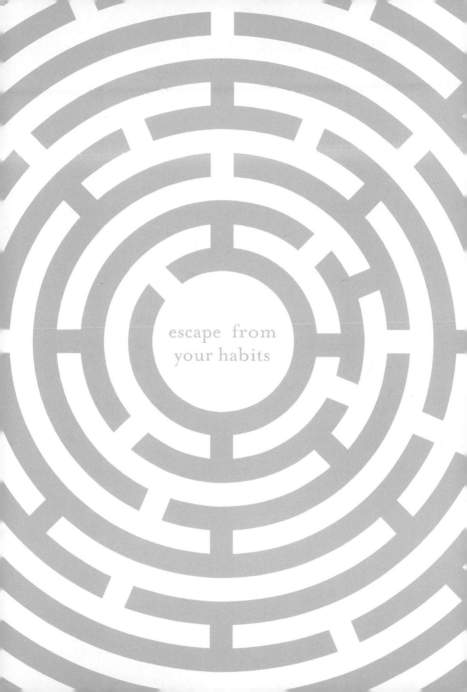

escape from
your habits

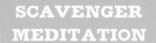

SCAVENGER MEDITATION

You will need:
One shoebox (or something similar).
Some paperclips. A snack (you mightn't be back in time for tea).
That's it.

Switch off your phone (you don't want to be distracted). Tuck your shoebox under your arm and walk outside, close your eyes and focus on the sensations of breathing. Feel the ground beneath your feet.

Walk to your nearest park or piece of waste ground. Wander around, following idle curiosity.

What catches your eye? A pile of leaves? Fading flowers. Some rubbish? If you feel drawn to something in particular, how does it affect your breath? Does your heart speed up? Do you feel excited? Feel the years falling away.

If something looks especially interesting, touch it or pick it up. Peer at all of its nooks and crannies (you're a child, remember). What does it feel like? Rough, smooth, ridged, soft, slimy or slippery? Soak up the textures. Smell it. Fresh, musty, earthy or stinky? Use all of your senses to explore what you find; you can even listen to it (remember the sound of the sea in a seashell?).

Let the scavenging begin; collect five objects and put them in your shoebox. It doesn't matter what they are, they just need to resonate with you in some way, whether they be twigs, petals, coins or crisp packets.

Either now or later, take your objects and spread them out. What's their story? If you found a man-made object, what was it originally used for? Where was it made? Who made it? Can you imagine what their life was like? How did it reach the park or waste ground?

For natural objects, where did it grow? Which wildlife relied on it for food, shelter or protection? Spend some time engaging with each object in this fashion and placing it into a wider context.

Close your eyes. Breathe. Imagine the web of connections binding us all together. Humanity and nature. Nature and humanity.

Breathe. Be playful. Stay curious. Paperclip something you found on your scavenging trip to this page. It could be a rose petal, a bus ticket or a leaf. The choice is yours, but make it consciously.

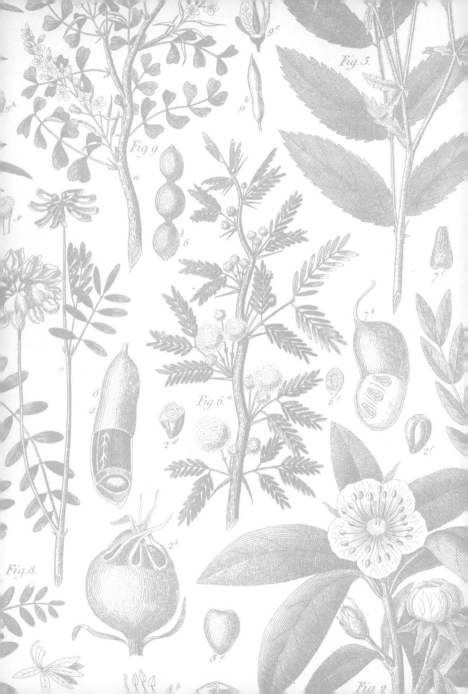

Fig. 9

Fig. 5

Fig. 6.

Fig. 8.

Fig. 2

seven: **AWARENESS**

*All that is solid melts into air**
* Apologies to Marx and Engels (they'd probably think meditation is
  a 'capitalist running-dog conspiracy'. It isn't, in case you were wondering.)

Thoughts, feelings and
emotions are created
by the body as much as
the brain. Even logic
and rationality are
profoundly influenced
by the body.

It ensures that you see the world as a reflection of yourself – rather than as objective reality.

Fancy a nice cup of tea?

If you want someone to like and trust you, give them a warm drink. Empathy and trust are warm.

If you're seeking a more masculine aura, give them something hard to hold. Masculine is hard.
If you want something to appear more valuable, make it heavy. Valuable is heavy.

Embodied cognition is the body's shorthand. It summarises and simplifies so you can make quick decisions in a complex and rapidly changing world.

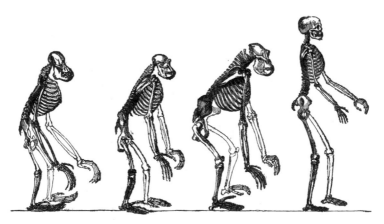

Unluckily, embodied cognition can lock you into negative spirals that lead to anxiety, stress, unhappiness and exhaustion.

A fleeting moment of stress creates tension in the body. The brain senses this physical tension and interprets it as stress. The body tenses a little more, breathing becomes a little shallower. The brain feels a little more stressed.

It's a downward spiral.

The same holds true for many other states of mind. The mind is reflected in the body – and the body in the mind. So states of mind and body can all feed back off each other in complex and unexpected ways.

When you think about it it's amazing that we're as sane and well balanced as we are.

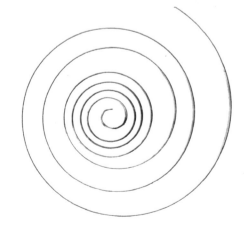

But, luckily, we have this magical thing called consciousness.

It allows you to see the interconnections between your mind and body, and releases you from negative and reactive states of mind.

So instead you can learn to *respond* rather than react.

And such awareness is only ever a single breath away.

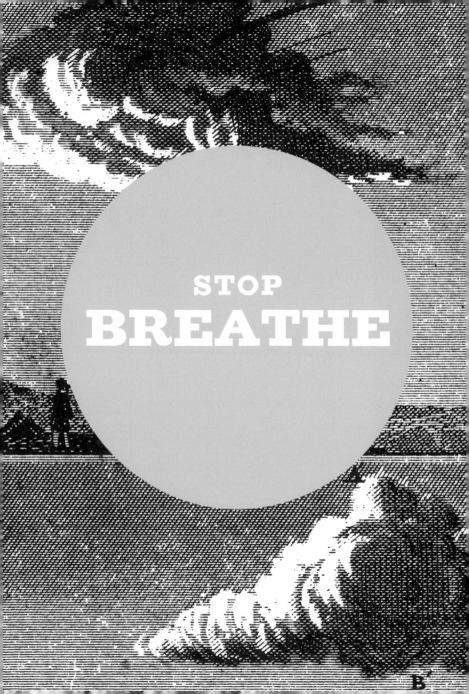

Mindful breathing teaches you that your most powerful states of mind are reflected in the body as physical sensations.

Be aware of these sensations. Each one is a message.

If you ignore them, or suppress them, then they will become ever more insistent and distressing until you can resist them no longer.

It's one of the most powerful sources of unhappiness and distress.

But there is an alternative.

If you consciously listen to these messages by actively feeling them in your body then something miraculous can happen. You'll realise that they rise and fall like the waves on the sea or your breath in your body.

And before long they'll begin to melt away of their own accord, leaving behind a calmer, happier, and more insightful mind.

Listen to
your body.

Listen
to your
breathing.

Become aware of your
stress and watch it dissolve.
Begin by tuning into your breath.
Feel its rise and fall. After a minute
or so, begin paying attention to
your body and locate where your
unpleasant feelings or emotions
have taken root.

Stress might be found as
tightness in your chest, shoulders
or neck. Anxiety as twitchiness
in your hands, legs or stomach.
Unhappiness as heaviness in your
face. It doesn't matter where they
are to be found, simply tune into
them and explore how they feel.

Do the sensations feel
'tight', painful or achy? Or
perhaps 'loose', exciting,
weak, or fleeting? It doesn't
matter how they feel. Simply
explore what you find.

When you realise that your mind has wandered, gently refocus your awareness back on the breath for a few moments, then begin exploring the physical feelings once again.

Notice how they rise and fall. Consciously feel them for a minute or so before mentally breathing into them. With each breath, does their intensity rise before falling away again? Notice how their patterns begin to change and then start to dissolve.

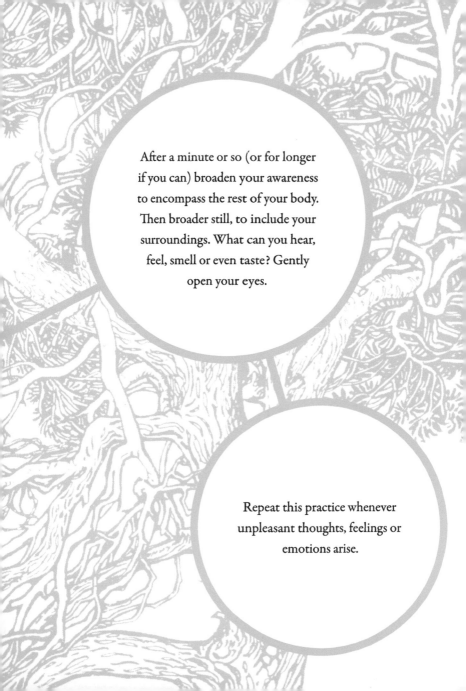

After a minute or so (or for longer if you can) broaden your awareness to encompass the rest of your body. Then broader still, to include your surroundings. What can you hear, feel, smell or even taste? Gently open your eyes.

Repeat this practice whenever unpleasant thoughts, feelings or emotions arise.

Mindfulness is
the observation
and acceptance of
your wandering
thoughts.

Whatever happens,
always remember
that you cannot fail
at meditation.

MINDFULNESS IS OBSERVATION WITHOUT CRITICISM

When you are meditating, try not to set yourself a definite goal, such as clearing your mind of thoughts or aiming to become happier or more peaceful or content.

These are often happy by-products of meditation. But if you aim for them, you will miss.

It may seem like an annoying paradox, but it is also true.

When you meditate, you find what you find.

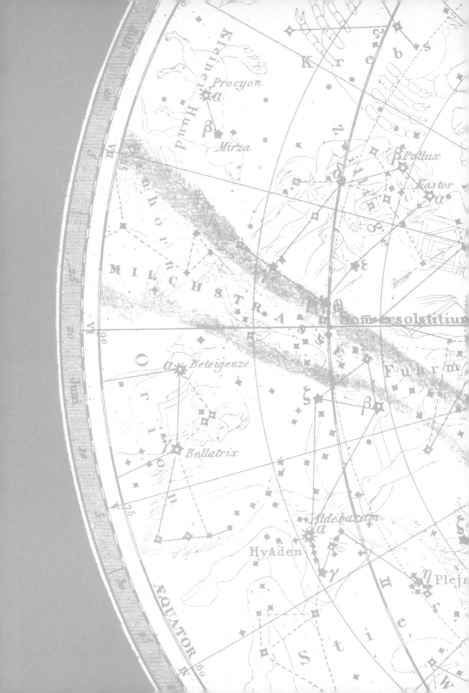

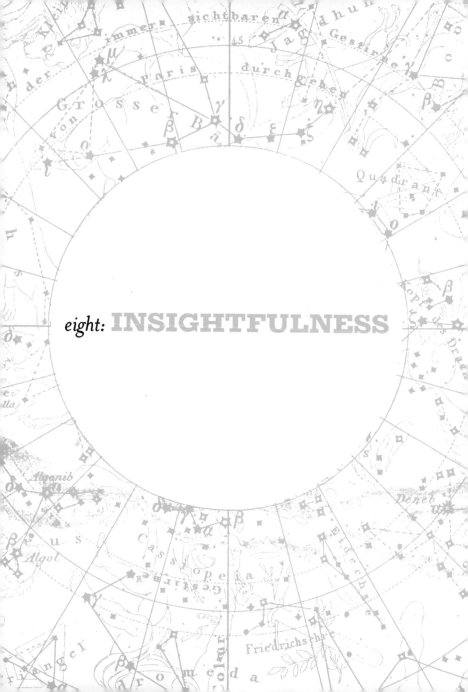

eight: **INSIGHTFULNESS**

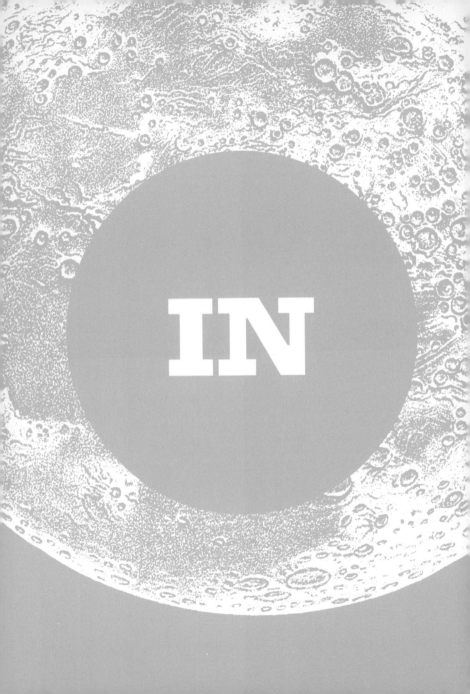

Our planet begins drawing her breath in May.

For months, global oxygen levels have been falling
and carbon dioxide concentrations rising.

Then something miraculous happens – the sun
crosses an invisible threshold, triggering the vast forests
and grasslands of the Northern Hemisphere to set leaf
and bloom.

As they turn green and photosynthesise, they start
sucking unimaginable quantities of carbon dioxide
out from the atmosphere and releasing oxygen as
a by-product.

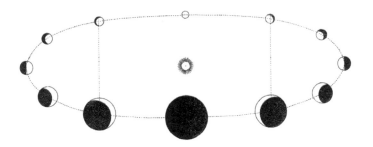

It begins almost overnight and accelerates rapidly. The northern Spring races forth at forty-five miles a day and then turns into summer.

The Earth's in-breath lasts for five months.

There's a brief pause.

Before autumn arrives and winter rushes in. Leaves begin to fall and grass to wither. As they break down, they consume oxygen and return vast quantities of carbon dioxide to the atmosphere.*

* These cyclical atmospheric changes are driven largely by the vast temperate forests and grasslands of the Northern Hemisphere. Take a look at this beautiful NASA video via www.franticworld.com/breathing

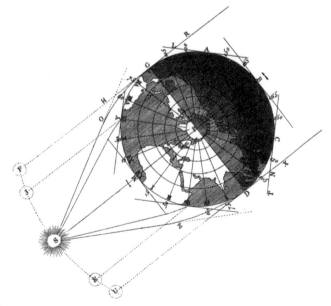

OUT

Elements of every breath you take
have been breathed by every person
in history.

Einstein, Shakespeare, Leonardo da Vinci.

Molecules from those breaths are still swirling
through the air, being inhaled and exhaled, becoming
incorporated into our bodies, turned into flesh and
bone, into other animals, plants, and rocks.

Wisps of those breaths first arose billions of years ago,
inside exploding stars.

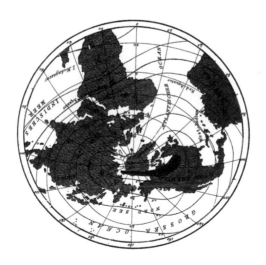

Stars draw their first breath when vast swirling clouds of hydrogen in deep space begin to condense. They become hotter, denser, until ...

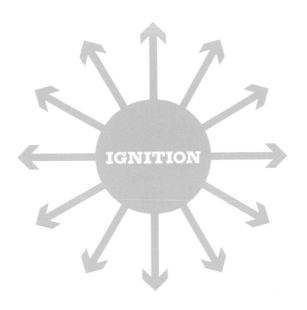

...the immense heat and pressure inside the stars foment a vast, uncontrollable, run-away nuclear reaction that continues for billions of years.

The stars twinkle and shine.

The star explodes in a supernova, showering the galaxy
with the elements needed for planets to form,
for an atmosphere to be created and for life to evolve.

Every molecule of the air you breathe, every atom in
your body, was born inside an exploding star billions of
years ago.

You needn't be a mystic to have mystical moments ...

... just a basic knowledge of physics.

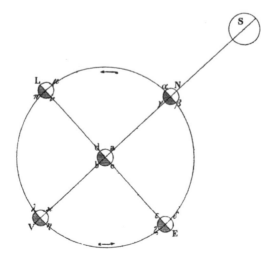

TIME TO TAKE A BREATHER...

Go outside on a starry night. Take off your shoes and socks. Feel the ground beneath your feet.

Look upwards.

Breathe.

See the stars streaming off into infinity in every direction. Not just unimaginably big but true, never-ending, ever expanding, infinity.

Focus on your breath as it flows in and out. Feel the soles of your feet touching the ground, the cool night air washing over you.

Feel the stillness, the expectation, infinity itself...

Look at the stars as they twinkle. Those twinkles may have taken billions of years to reach you.

Breathe.

Love, love
the arriving
of the light …

Breathe.

Our universe first appeared as a 'singularity': a point of infinite energy and density that erupted out of nothingness.

A fluctuation in emptiness.

Space and time tore out from this at near-infinite speed.

One 'moment' there was nothing. The next, everything.

An exhalation, if you like.

The universe will begin its end when space and time cease to expand.

Everything will pause for a while .

And then begin racing back to a singularity at an ever accelerating pace.

An inhalation, if you will.

For centuries, people have prepared their mind with a very special breathing meditation before contemplating such ideas.

The state of mind it engenders has countless other benefits too.

It enhances creativity and clarity of thought while promoting a sense of peace and well-being. It encourages a sense of wonder, of awe, of curiosity – the foundations of a happier and more meaningful life.

It soothes the inner critic and allows your true self to bubble through to the surface. It will give you the courage to accept yourself with all of your faults and failings. To treat yourself with the kindness, empathy and compassion that you truly need ... so you can look outwards and embrace the world.

And when you do this...

...you'll discover the secret to living mindfully.

INSIGHT MEDITATION

Sit.

Close your eyes and tune into the world around you, becoming aware of the space around you. You might hear some noise ... Whatever is there, pay attention to the sounds for a few moments.

Begin building up a picture of how your body feels, beginning with your feet. Pay attention to both feet simultaneously for a few moments. Tune into the sensations, then move your attention to the ankles ... the lower legs ... knees ... upper legs ... hips and pelvis ...

Take your time. There's no rush.

Move your attention to both hands...arms... shoulders... neck... head...face...nose... and lips.

Soak everything up, in turn, over a minute or so.

Pay attention to the movement of your breath in your body – follow it all the way in ... and all the way out. Don't try to change anything, just feel its natural flowing rhythm.

When you realise that your mind has wandered, watch the thoughts themselves. It doesn't matter whether they're in the form of words or pictures, simply pay attention for a few moments and then return to the breath.

After a couple of minutes, shift your awareness to any thoughts or emotions passing through your mind.

These thoughts and emotions – and the gaps in between them – will now become the focus of the meditation.

Don't force any thoughts to appear in your mind, simply wait patiently for them to arrive. Let the mind be completely free … free from any control or expectation.

Try to become aware of the moment that thoughts first appear, then watch them for a few moments. Notice how they rise and fall; how one thought triggers the next and the next.

Notice how thoughts tend to melt away when you stop reacting to them, when you stop judging or criticising them.

Notice what happens when your thoughts momentarily stop ... try to gain a sense of what it feels like ... try to gain a sense of what the absence of thoughts feels like.

It might feel like a place of pure tranquillity or it might feel like an emptiness or perhaps of something vast just beyond your grasp. Whatever it seems like, simply wait as if you're sitting on the edge of a vast pool. Waiting. Patiently ...

After a while you'll realise that your mind has wandered away with itself again. When you do so, gently shift your attention back to the breath, and after a few breaths begin waiting patiently for another thought or emotion to appear.

You may run through this cycle of mind wandering and refocusing countless times. It doesn't matter. What matters is paying attention to your mind with all of its toings and froings

Checking out.

After ten minutes or so, gradually begin to shift your attention to the world around you, becoming aware of the space around you. Open your eyes. Begin to move. See if you can maintain the essence of this clear-sighted awareness as you move through your day.

The Insight Meditation works best if you practise regularly. Ten or twenty minutes a day, four or five days a week is sufficient.

At the beginning of this book
you took a breath, maybe your first
conscious breath in years and
one of the most important breaths
you've ever taken.

Take a few moments to think
about how far you've come and
how the journey has already begun
to transform your life.

The art of breathing lies in having
the courage to let go. To let go and
allow your breath to breathe itself.
And when you do this, something
miraculous begins to happen, life
begins to live through you.

You become quicker to laugh and slower to anger, life becomes less frantic and exhausting, sleep more restful. You rediscover your sense of wonder, awe, and outright joy.

But most of all, you accept your imperfections with a warm smile rather than biting criticism.

Now breathe.

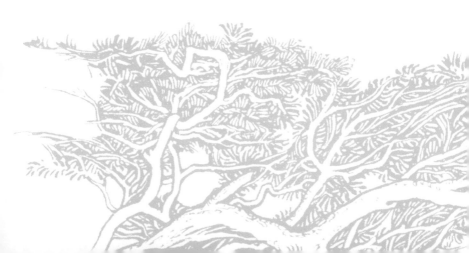

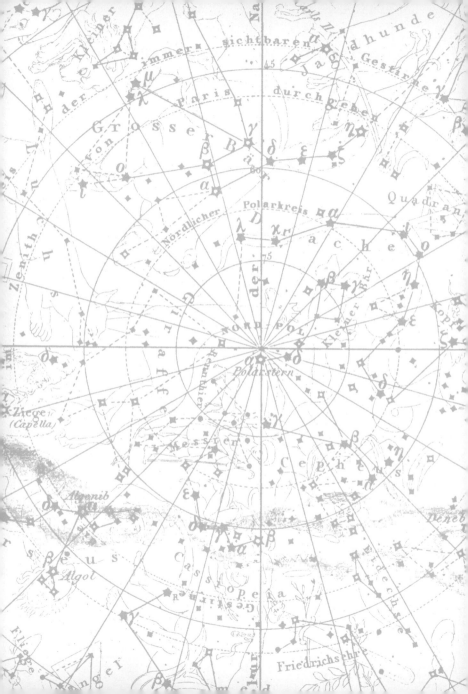

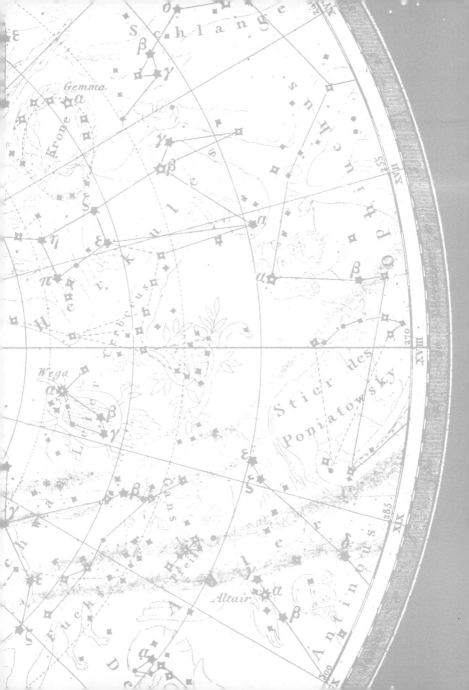

Dr Danny Penman is a qualified meditation teacher and an award-winning writer and journalist. He is co-author of the international bestseller Mindfulness: A Practical Guide to Finding Peace in a Frantic World. He has received journalism awards from the RSPCA and the Humane Society of the United States. In 2014, he won the British Medical Association's Best Book (Popular Medicine) Award for Mindfulness for Health: A Practical Guide to Relieving Pain, Reducing Stress and Restoring Wellbeing (co-written with Vidyamala Burch). His books have been translated into 30 languages. His journalism has appeared in the Daily Mail, New Scientist, The Independent, The Guardian, and The Daily Telegraph. He trained to teach mindfulness with the acclaimed Breathworks.

Acknowledgements

I am enormously grateful to Sheila Crowley at Curtis Brown. If you knew Sheila, you'd realise that she is quite simply the best agent and friend you could wish for. And thanks to Lisa Milton of HQ. She mentioned the title of this book and everything fell into place.... She's one of those rare people who is full of brilliant ideas. When we're together, you can't shut either of us up. Thanks also to Charlotte Mursell. She had the difficult task of reining me in and making sure that this book was finished on time. And thanks to Steve Wells who did the design and layout of this book. He's brilliant and I love his work! Thanks also to Louise McGrory of HQ for helping conceptualise the design with Steve.

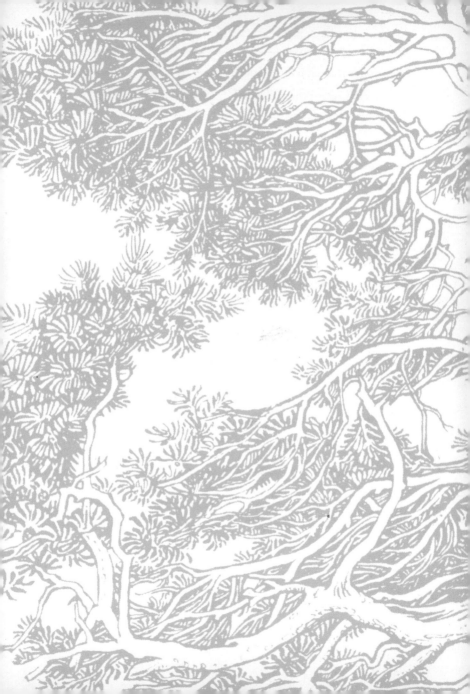